CP and ME

by Kirk & Emily Christensen

editing & design by Nathan Christensen

HWC PRESS

Hi!

My name
is Kirk!

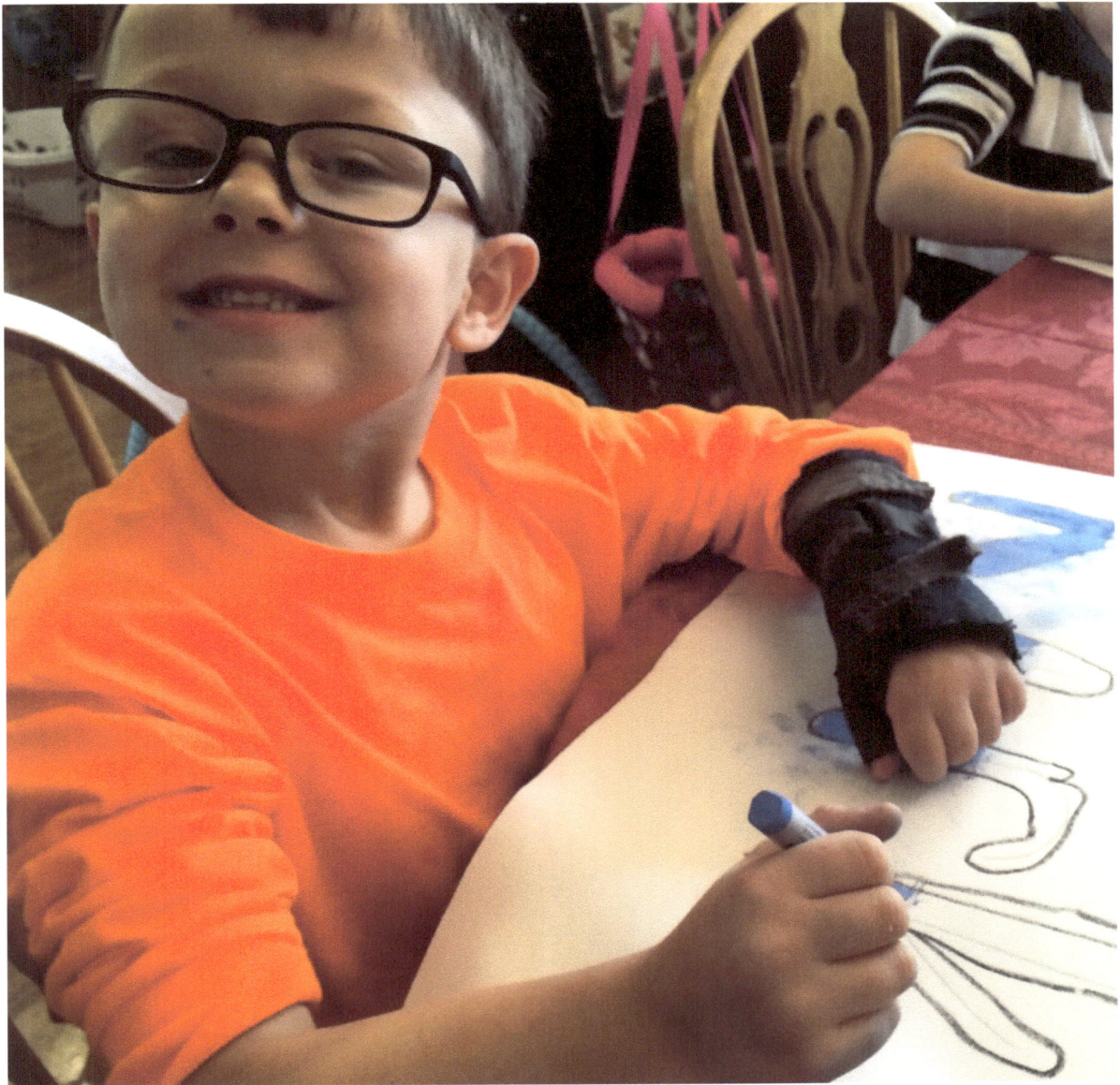

And this isn't a cast on my arm.

It's my brace.

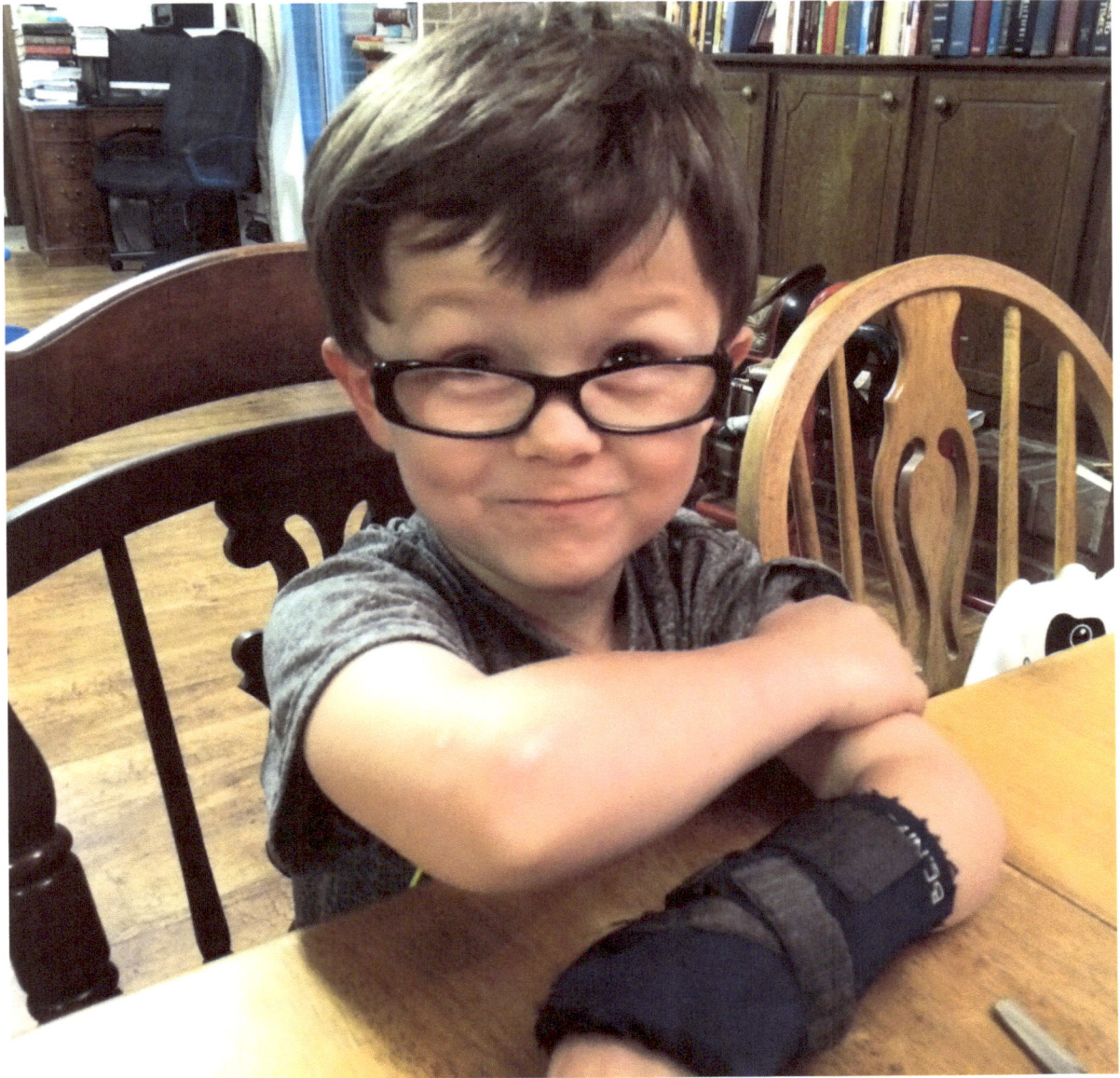

Because I have Cerebral Palsy.

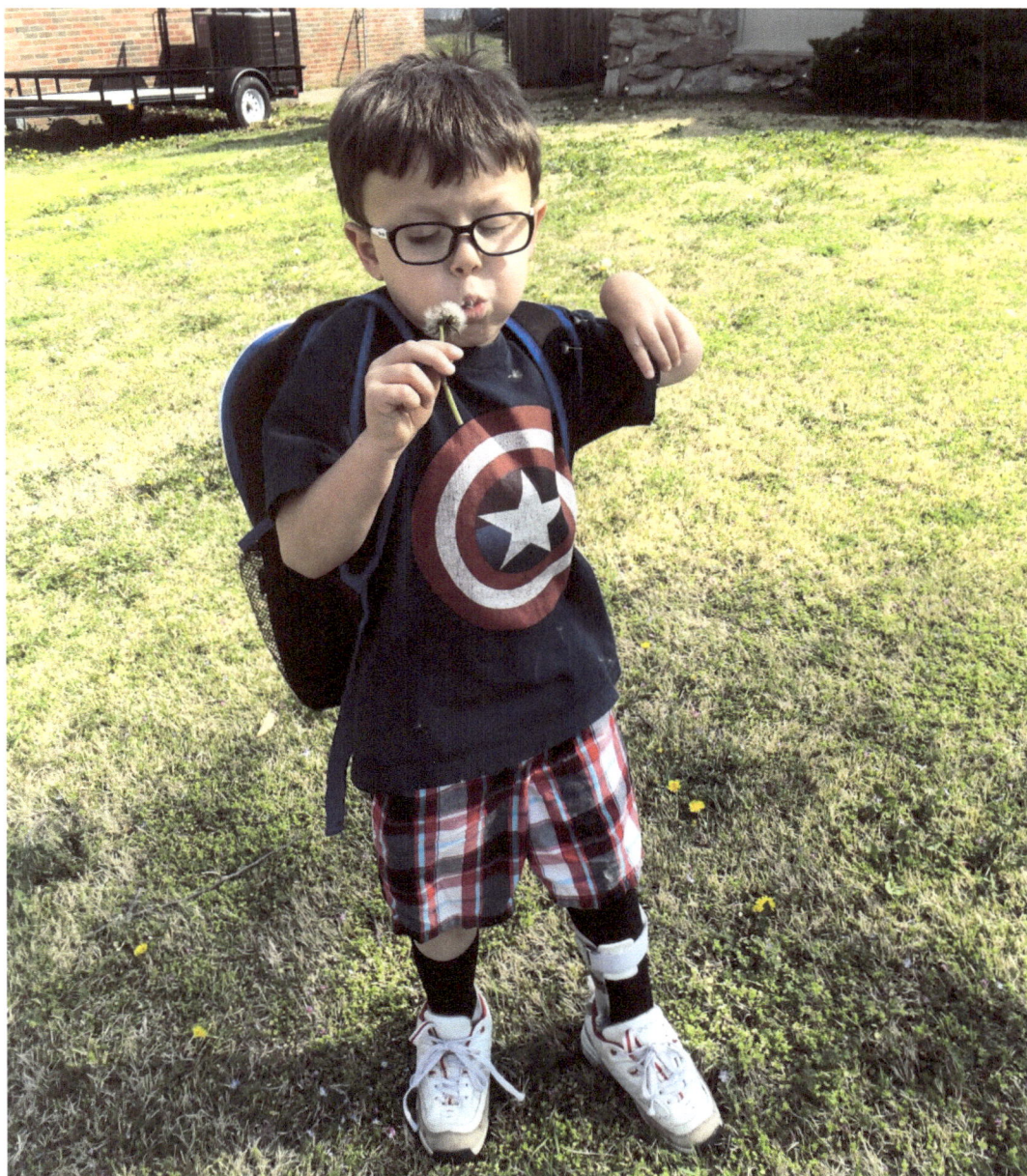

I have CP because I didn't get enough oxygen when I was being born.

I was about to die.

But I didn't. I survived.

For me, CP means my right hand is strong, but my left hand still helps.

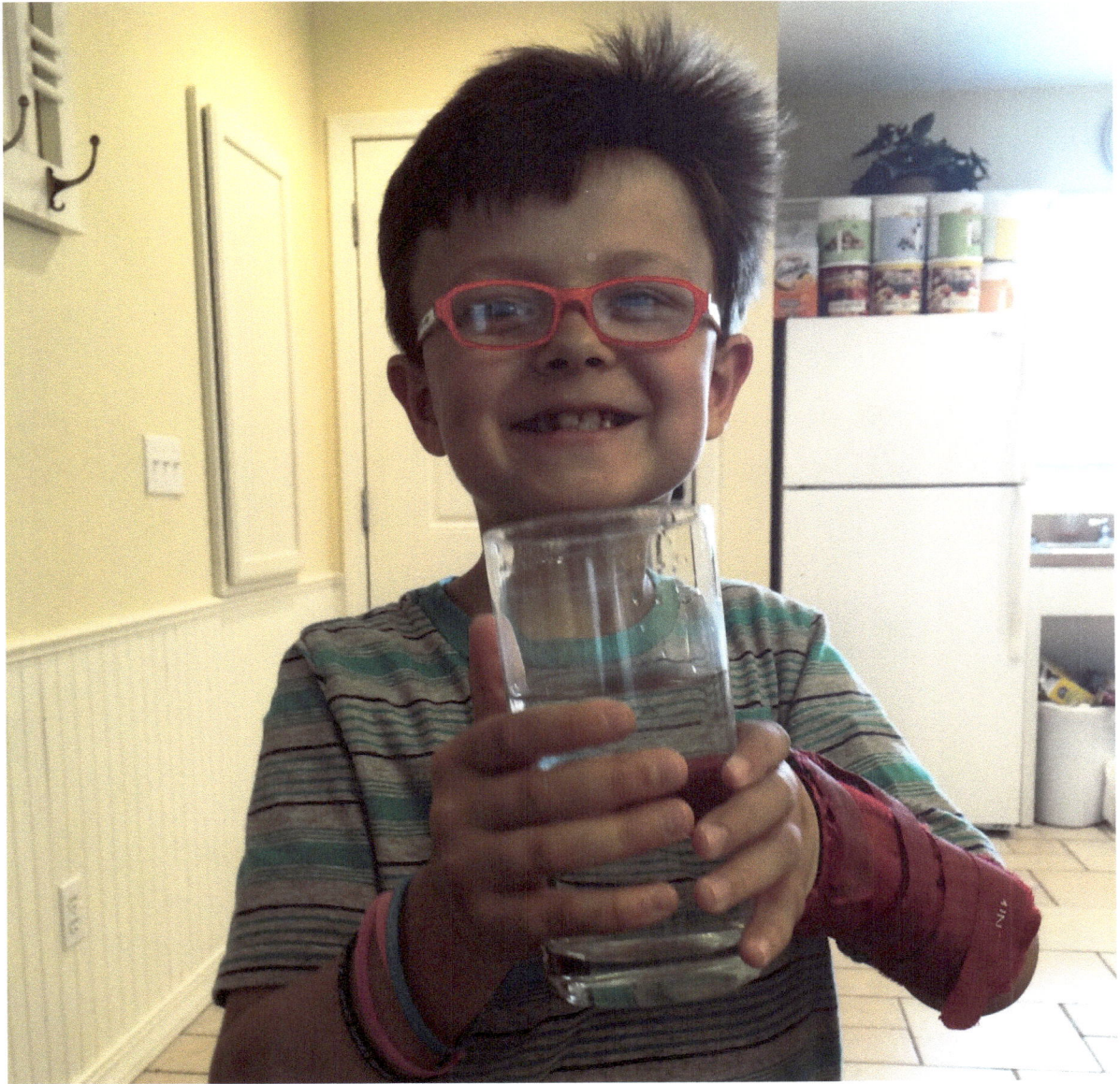

I also wear braces on my legs.

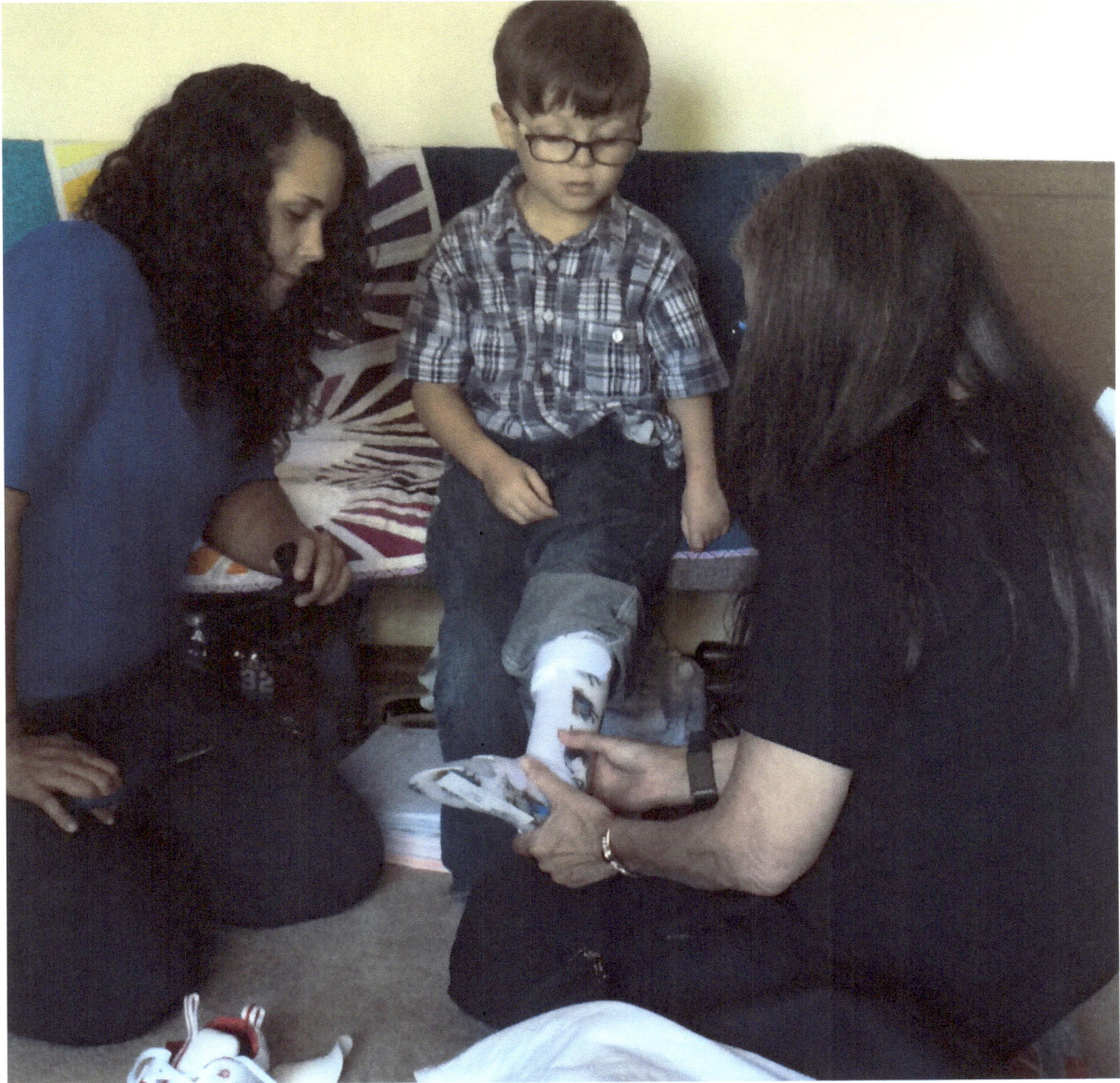

And I have a shunt in my head.

But you can't see it, even when my hair is cut.

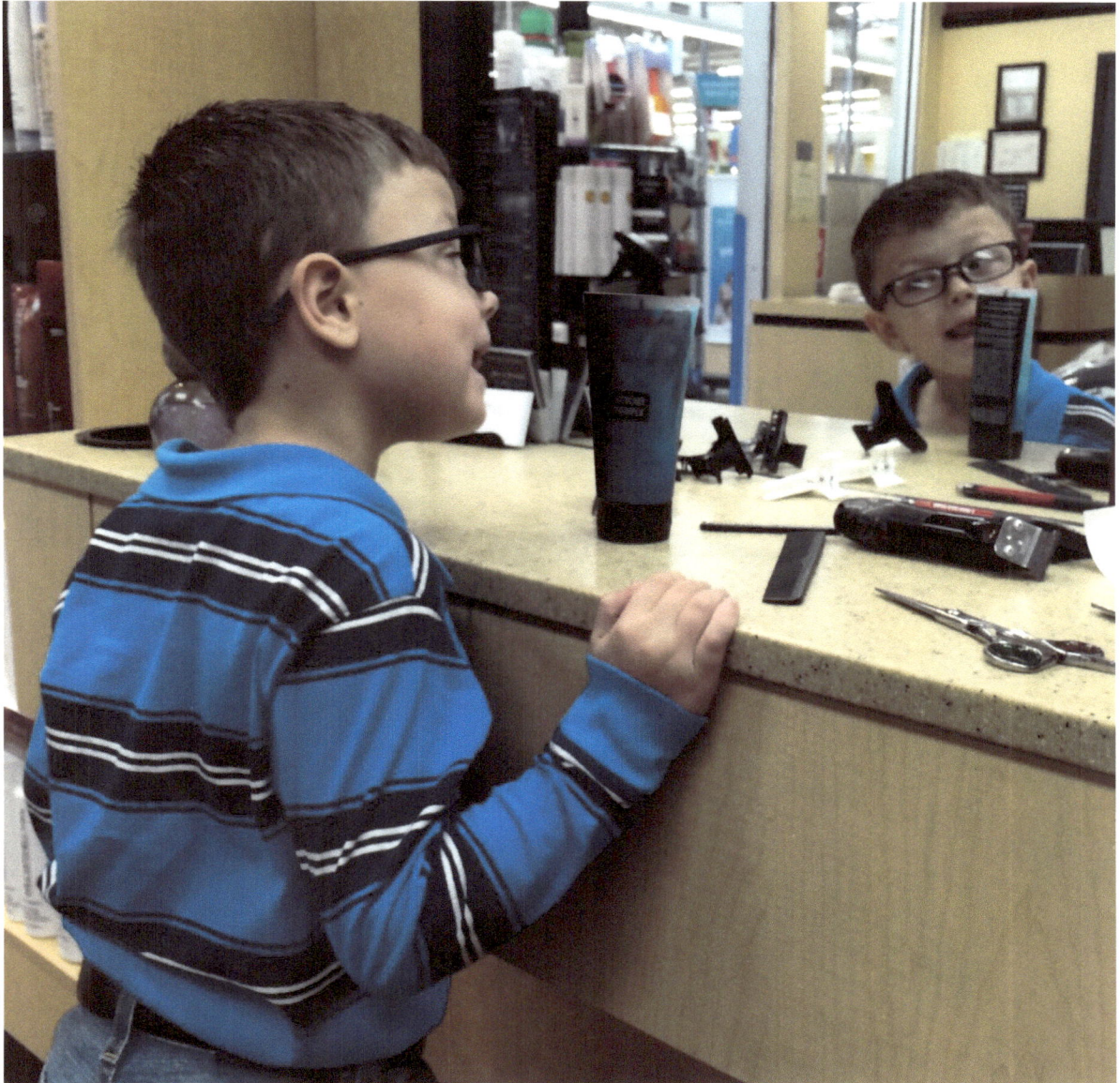

I used to have a feeding tube.

You can still see my awesome scars!

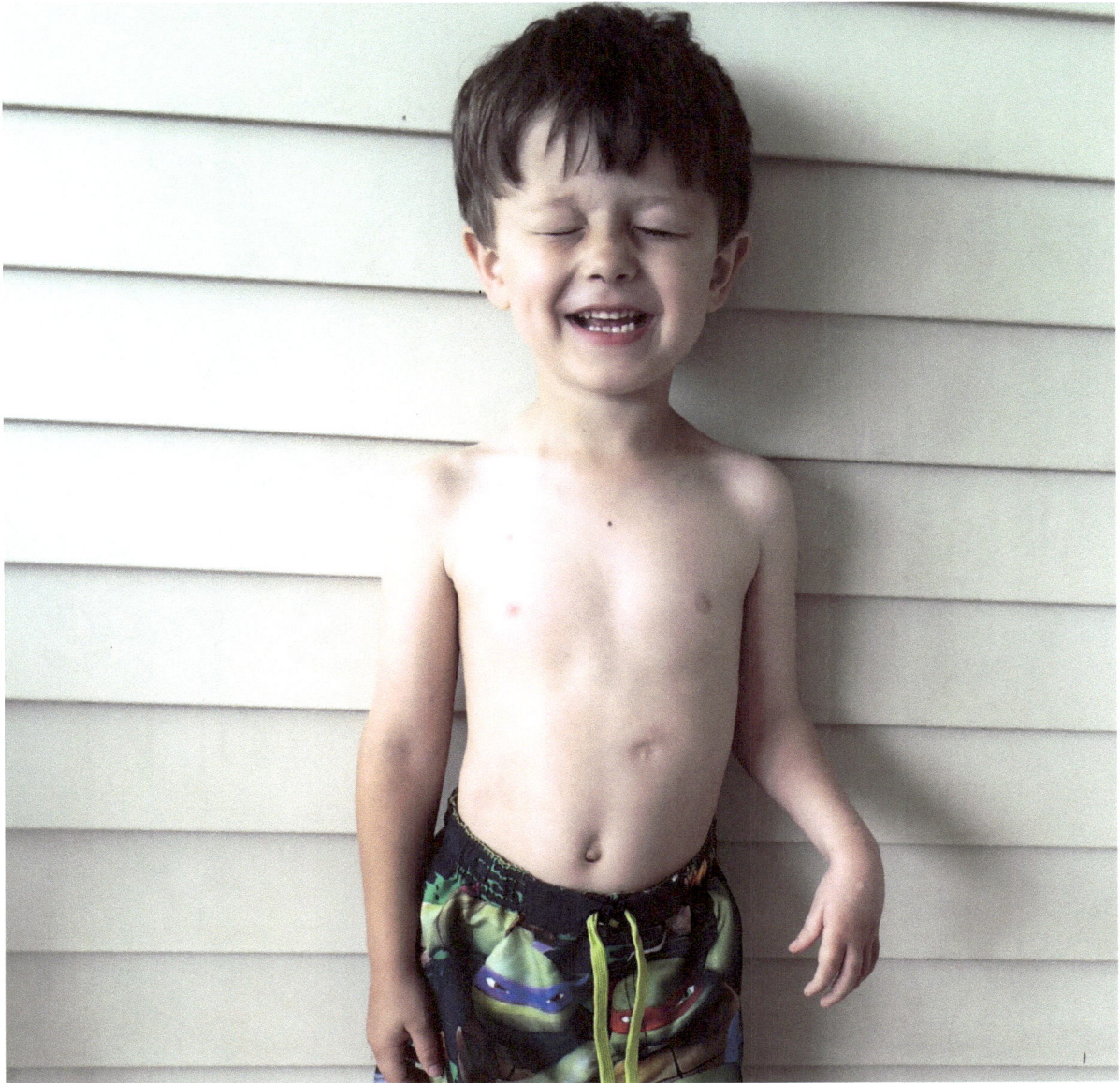

I have CP,
but CP isn't
what makes me
me!

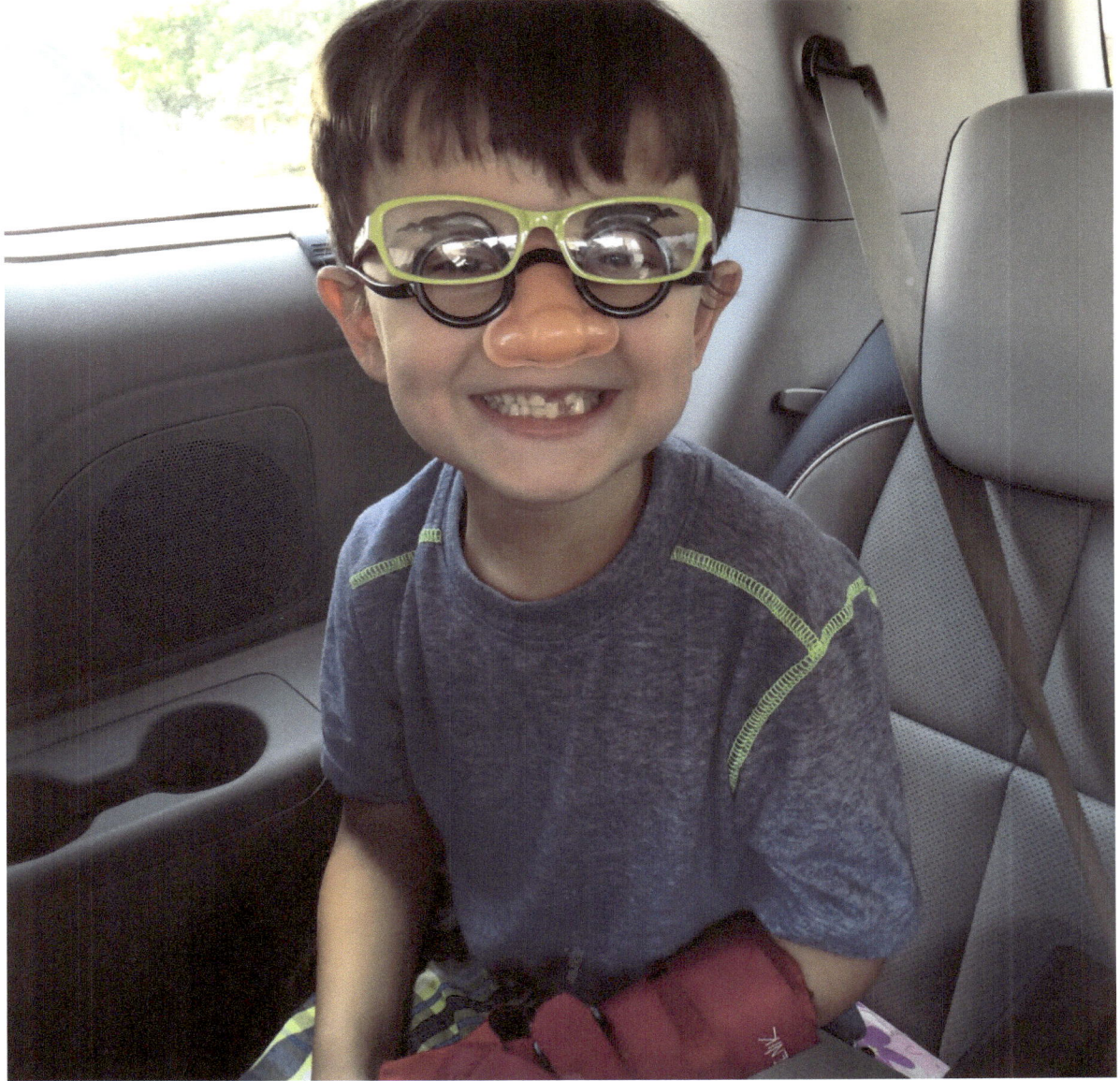

I climb.

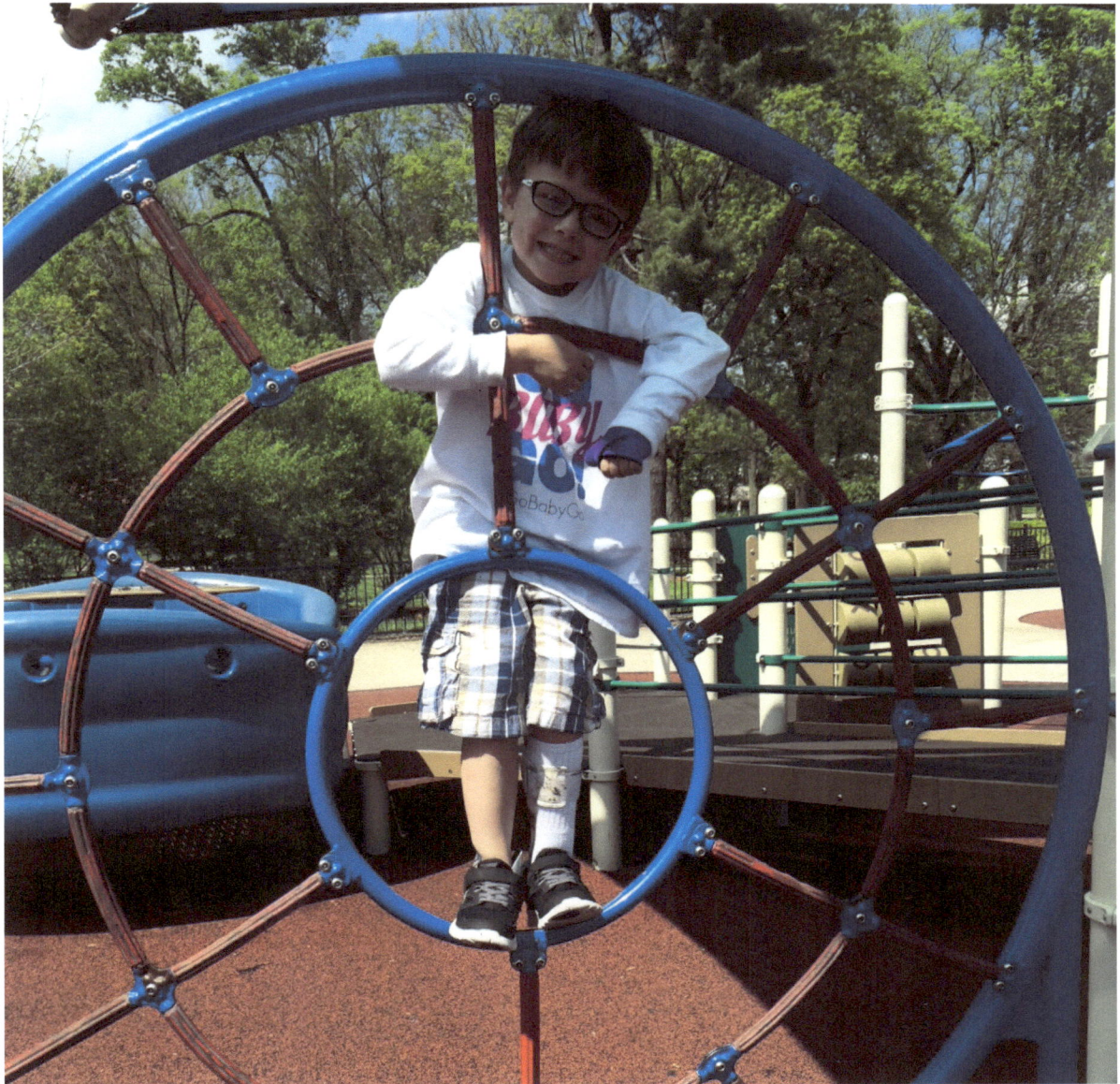

I study.

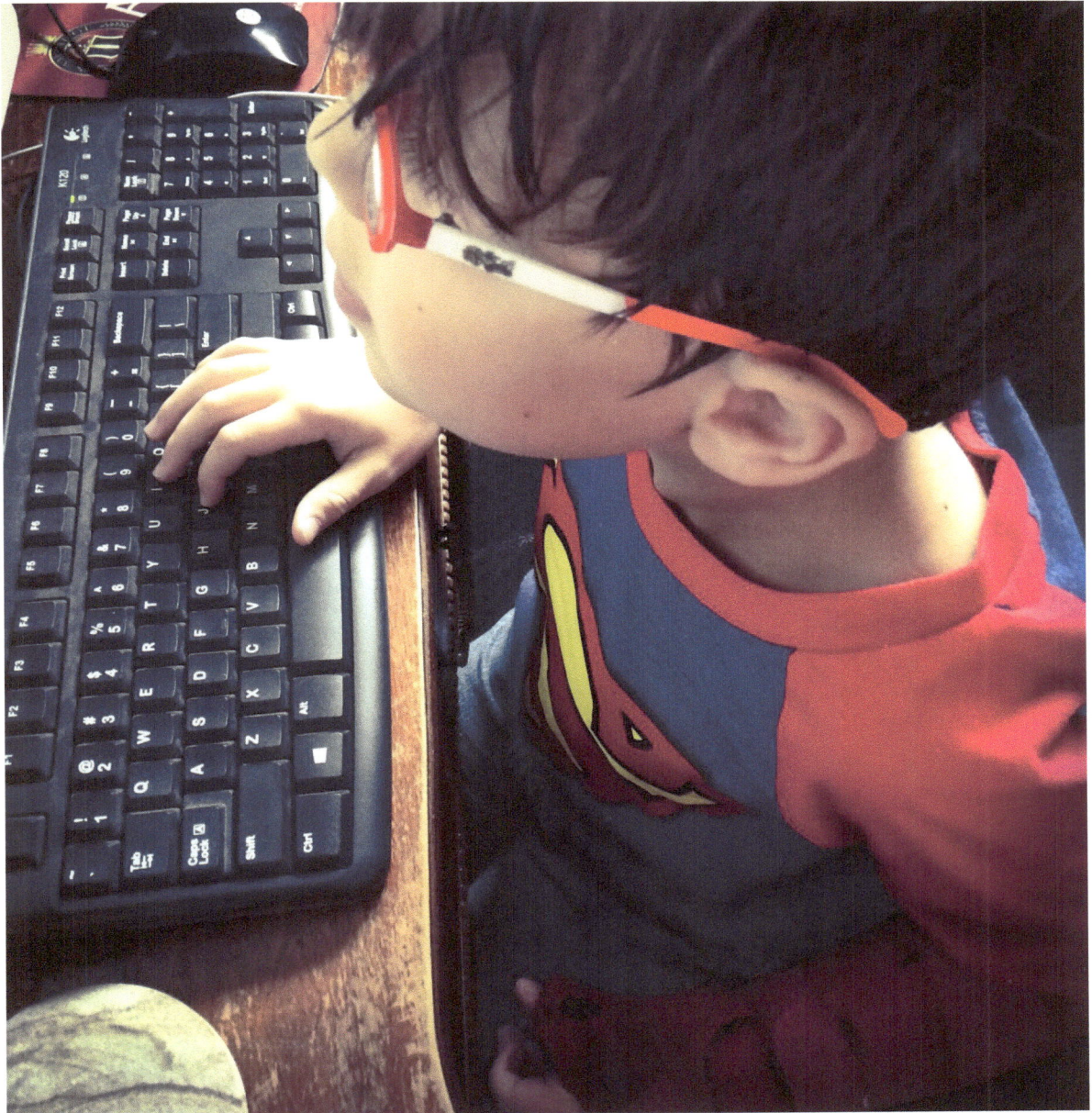

I build.

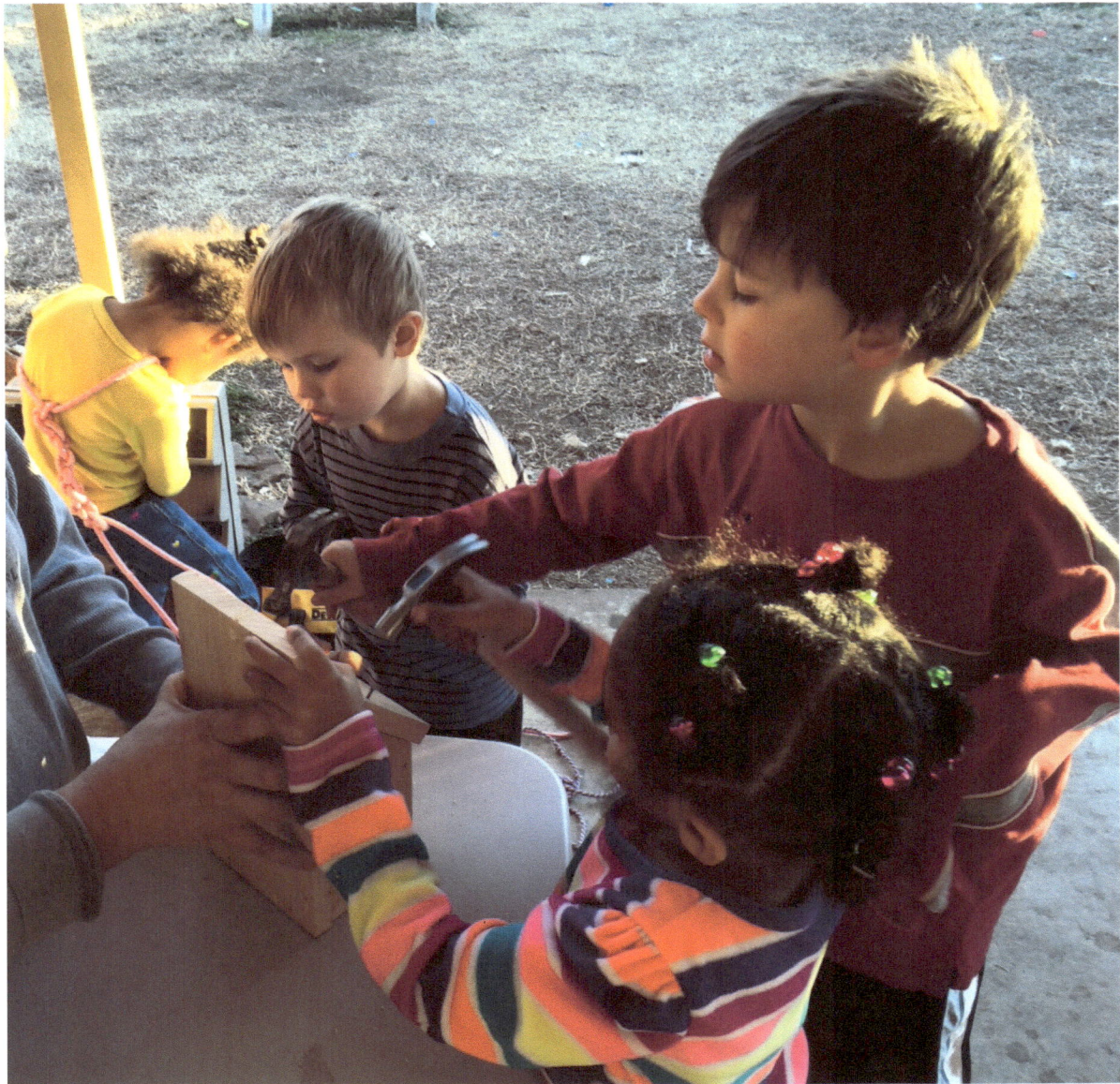

I splash.

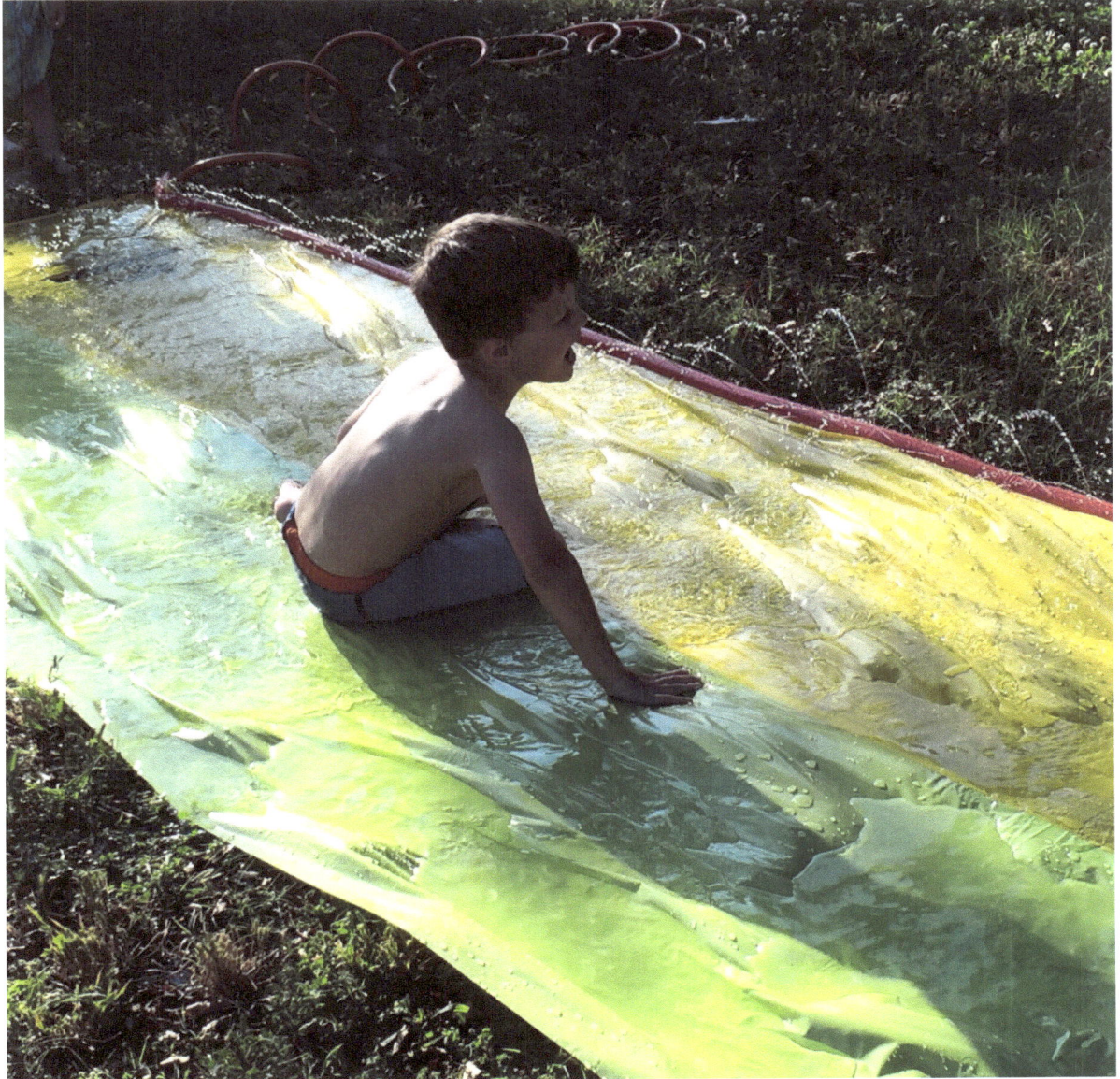

I jam.

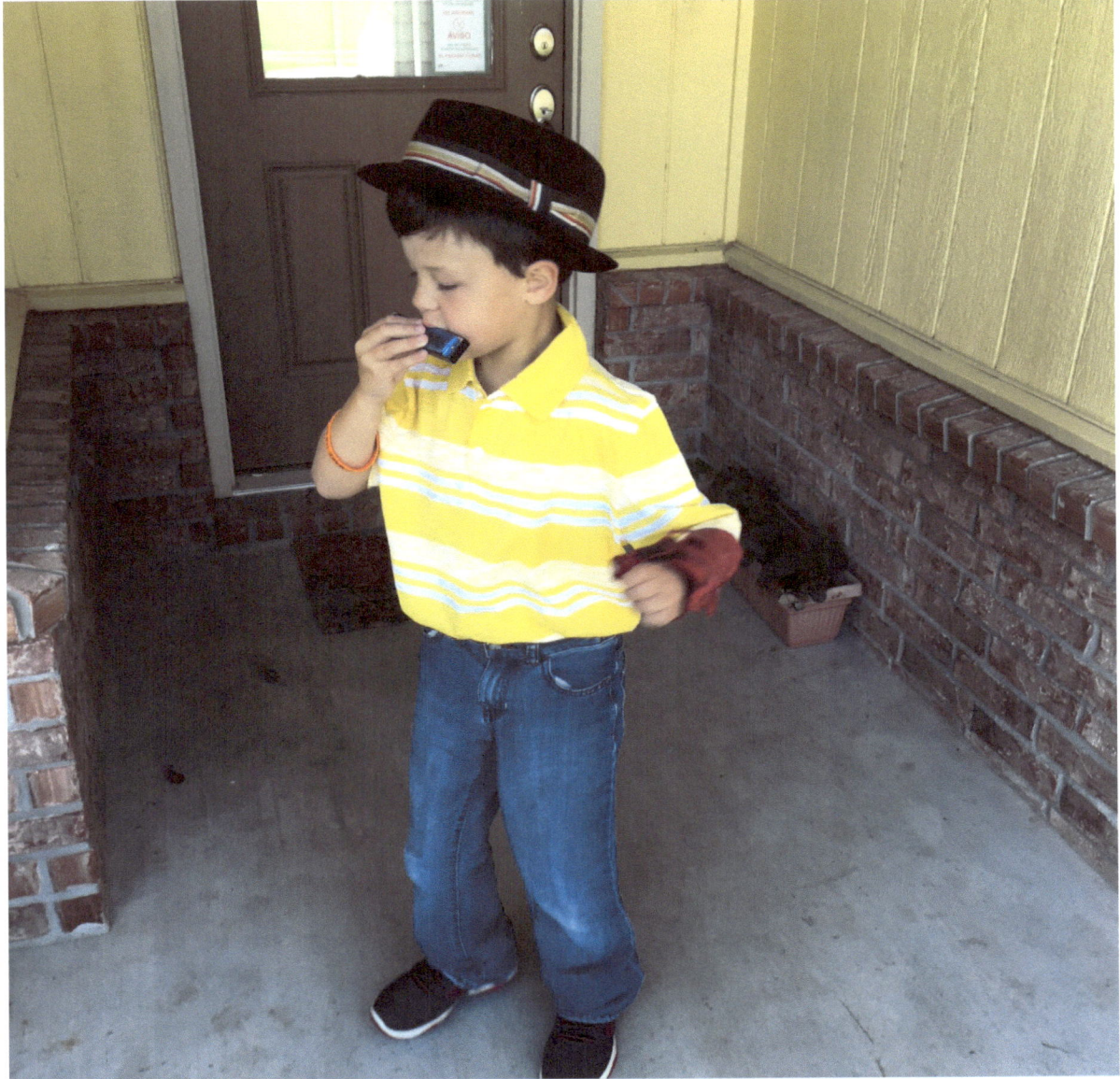

I roll.

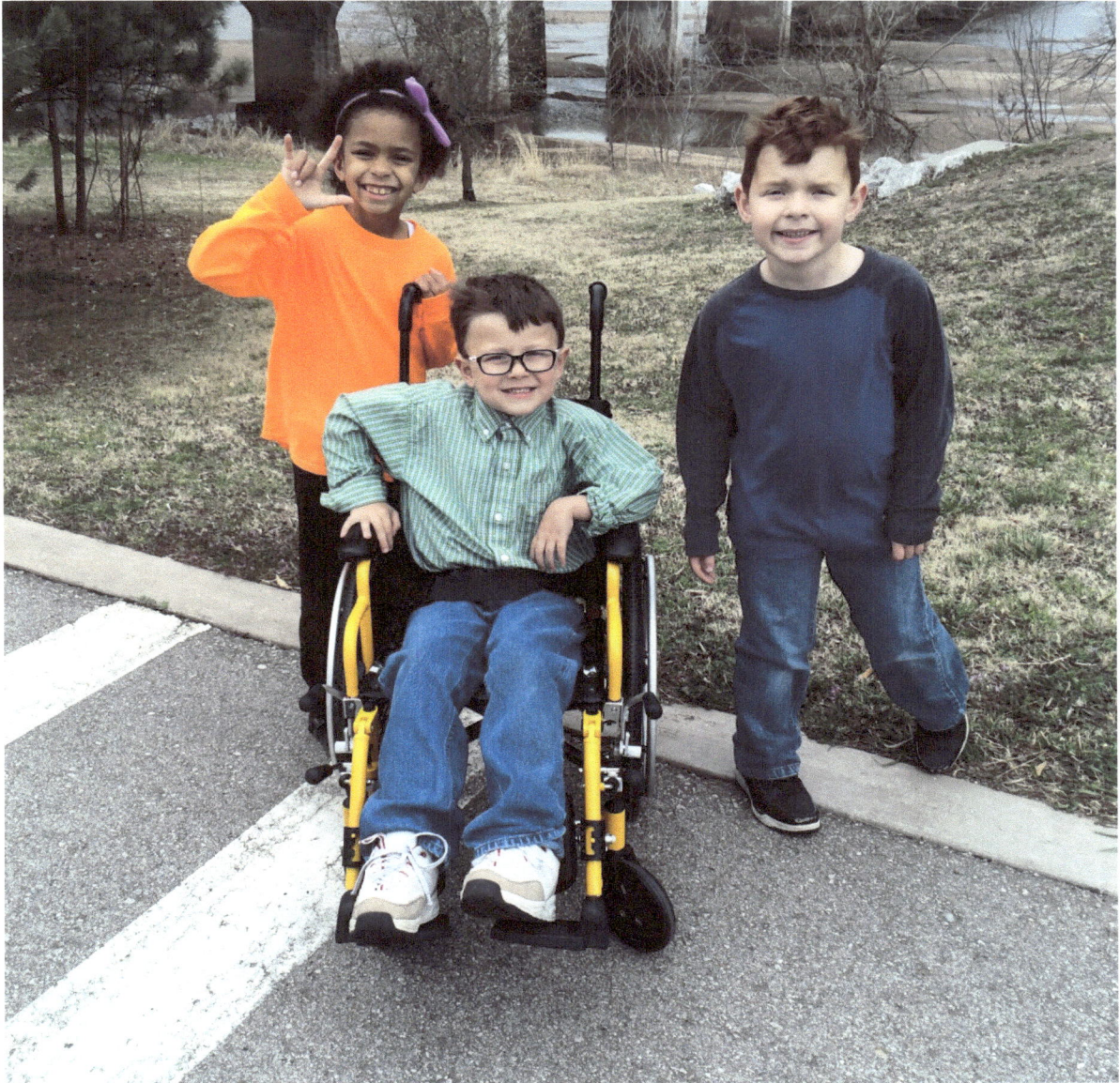

I defend
the universe.

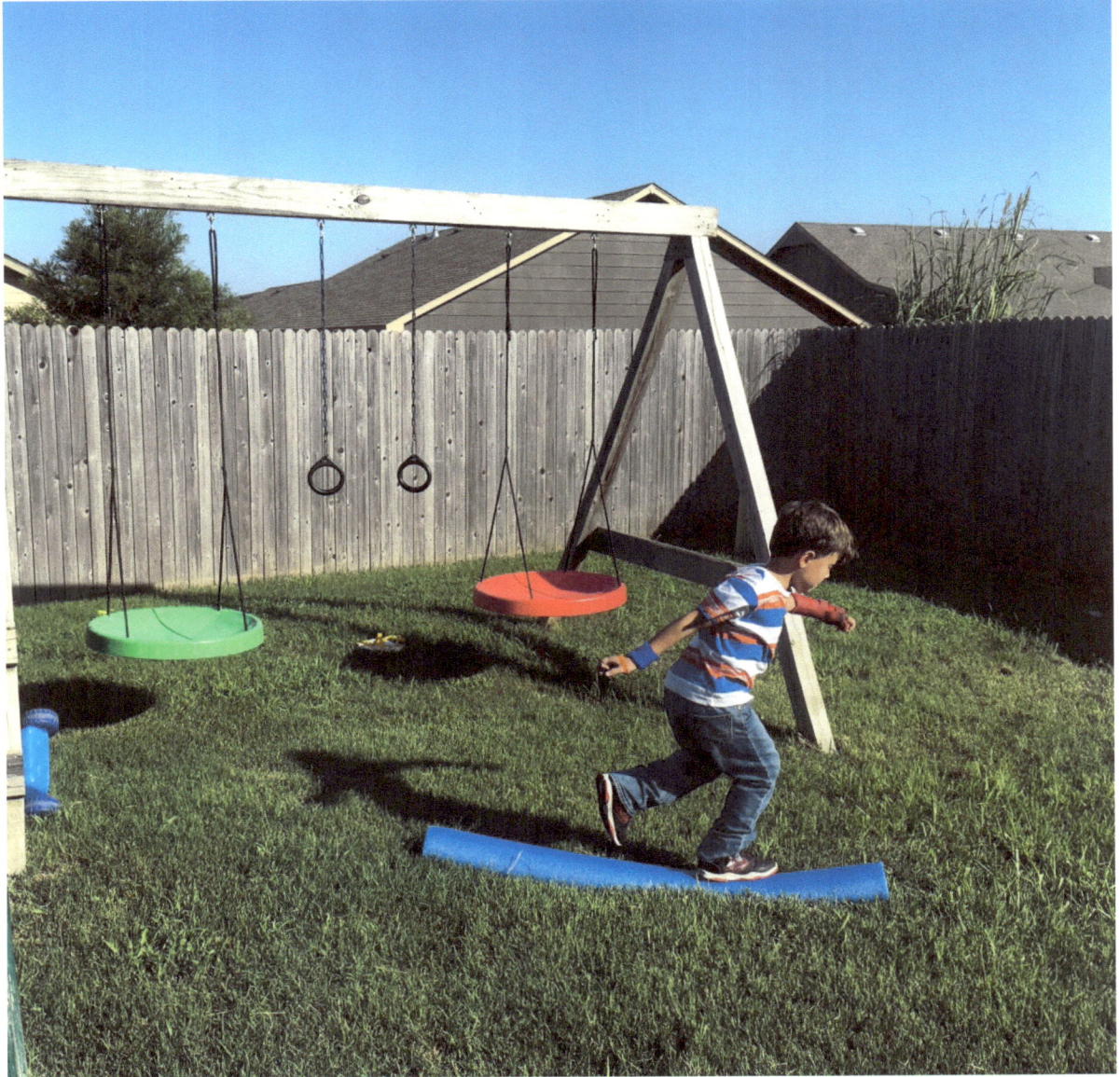

I have
good days.

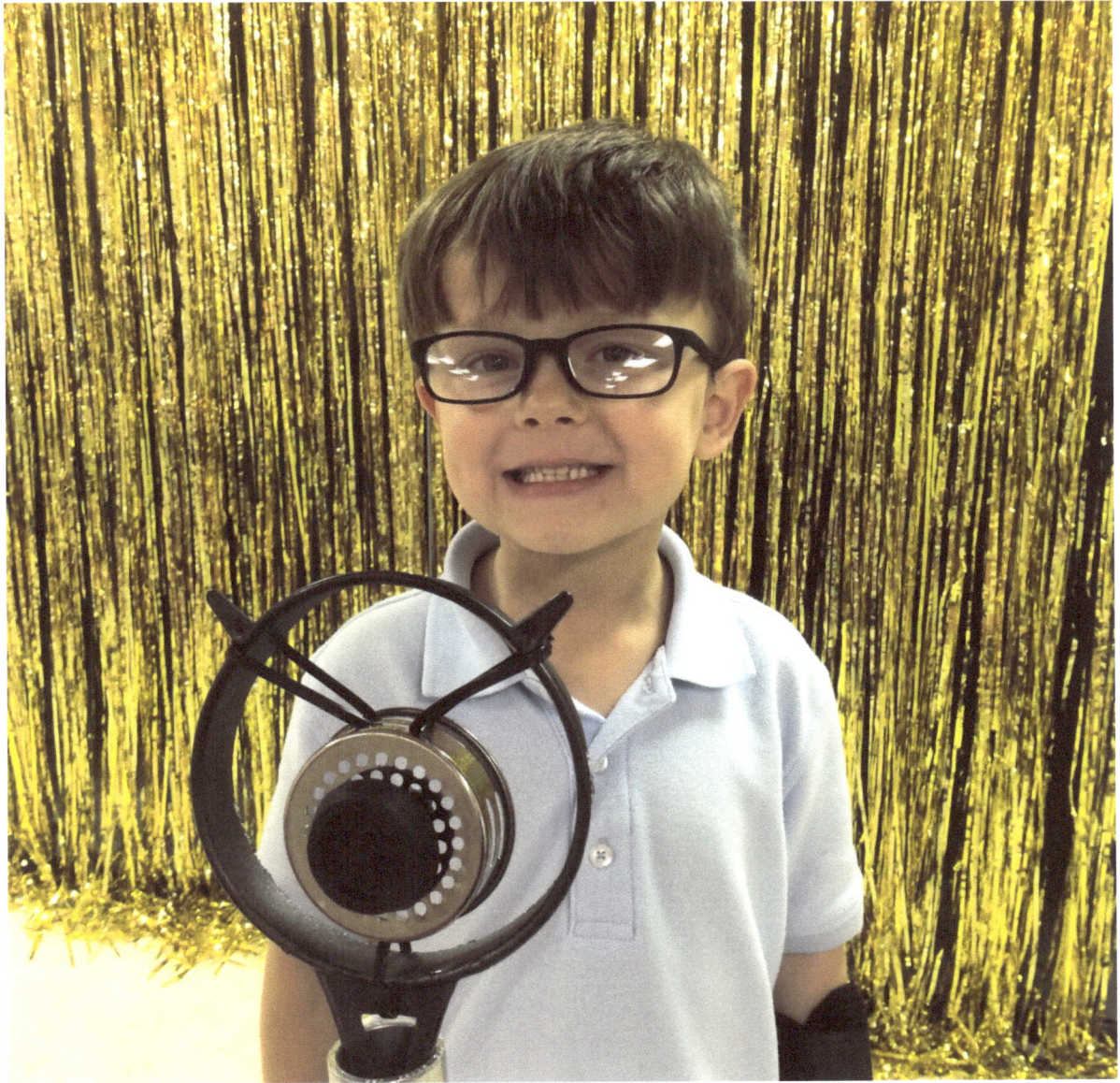

And I have
bad days.

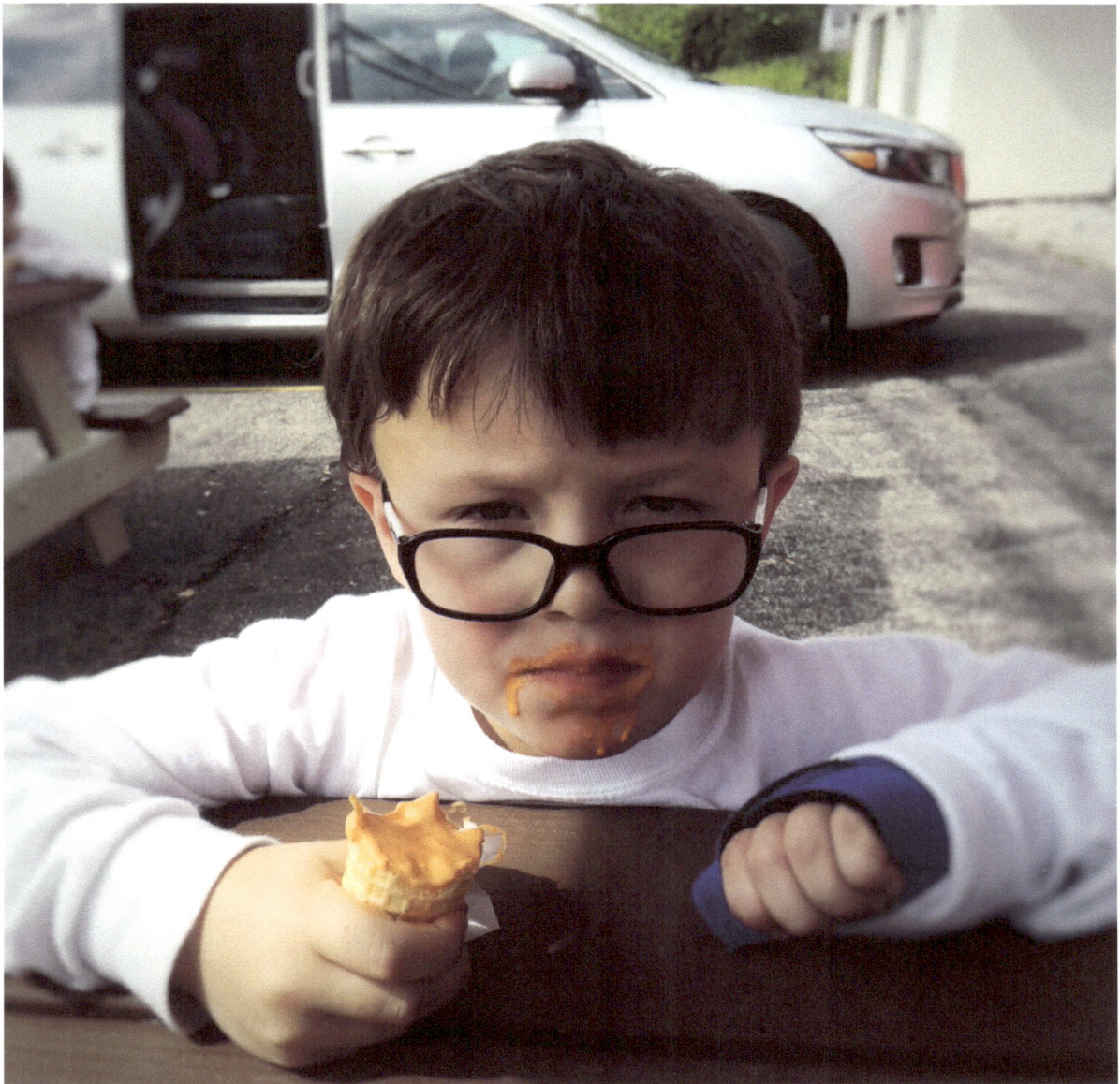

But nothing can stop me.

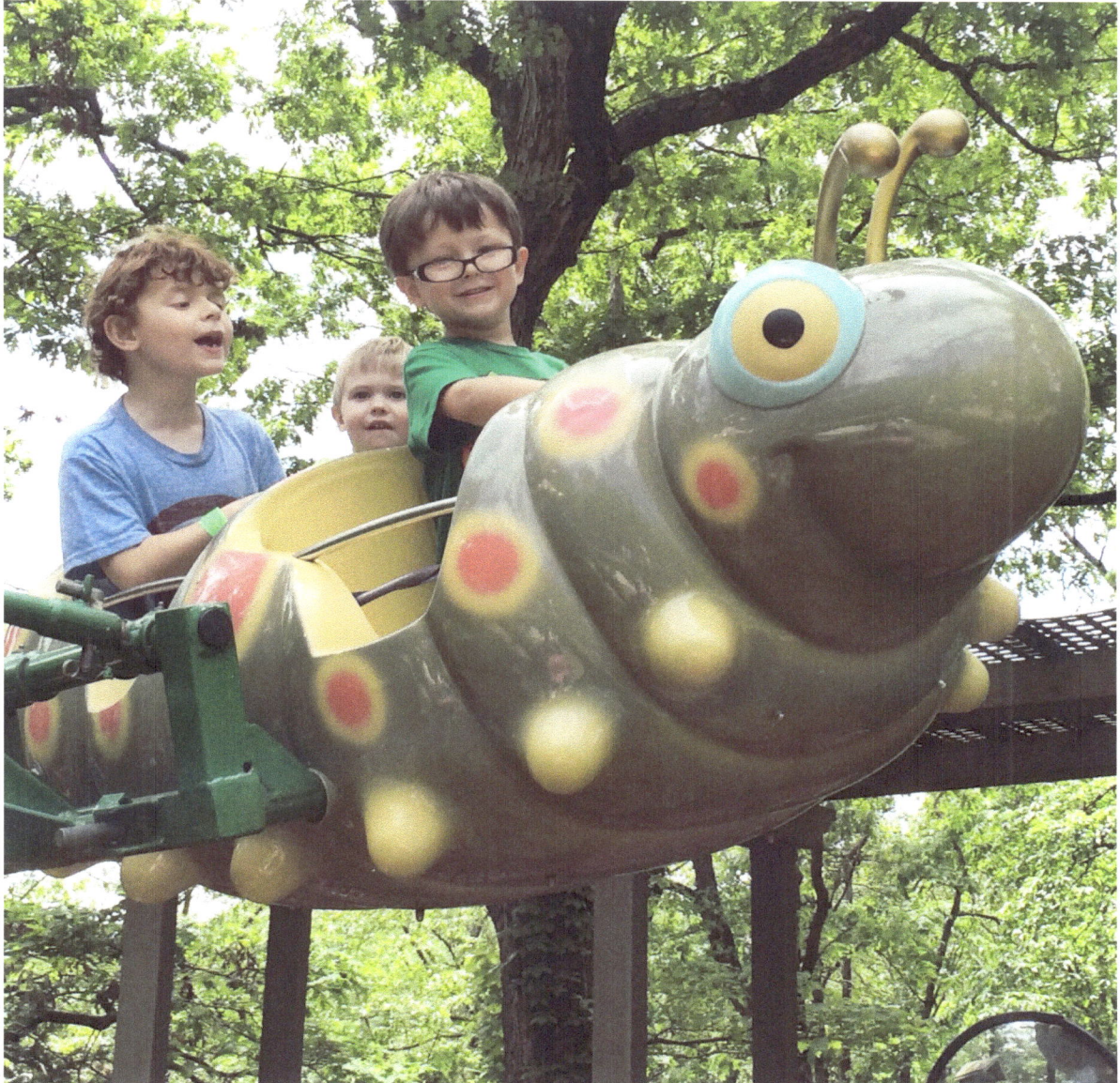

Because that's who I am.

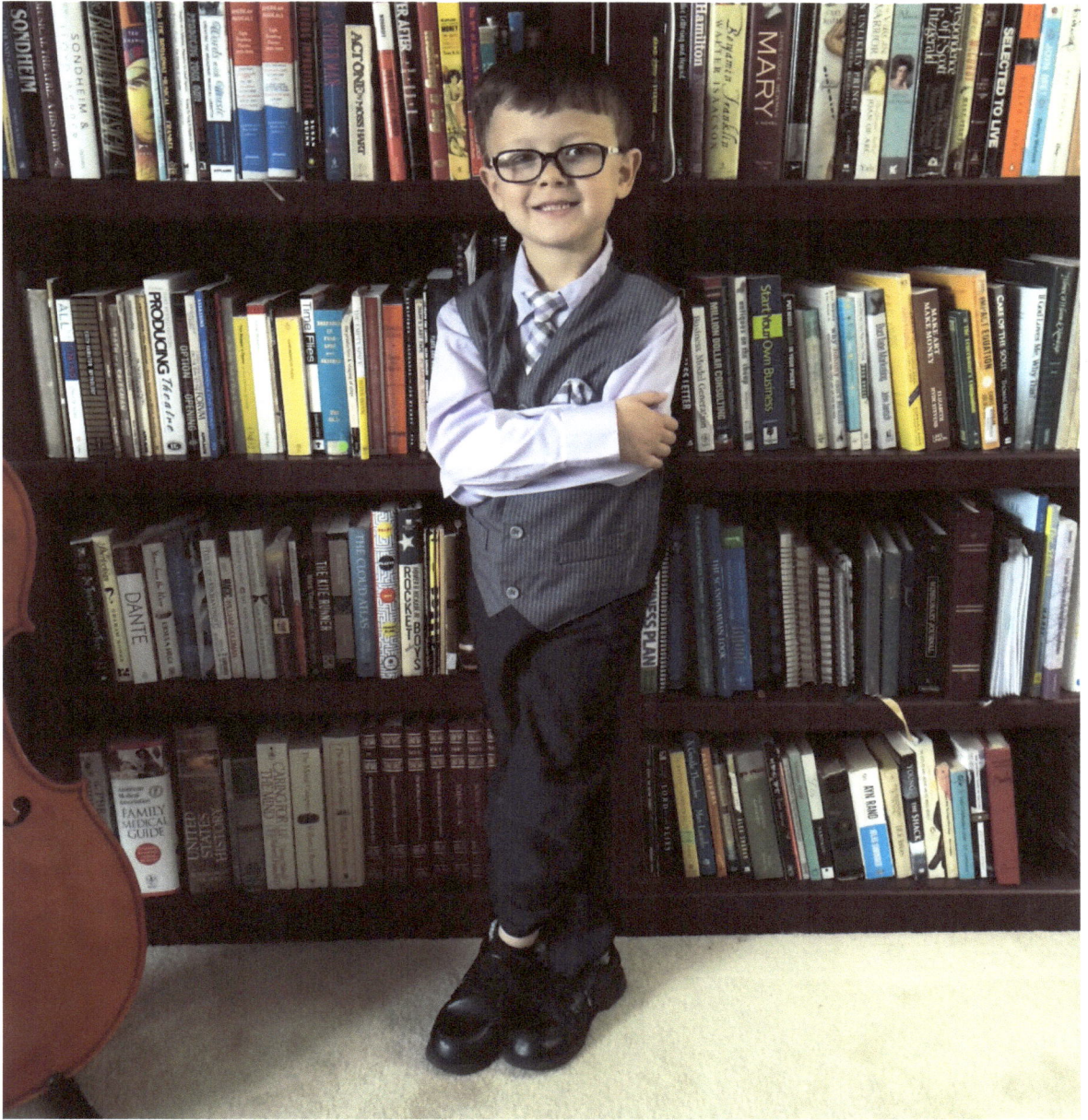

First Printing: 2017

ISBN: 978-0-9977588-6-3

HWC Press, LLC
P.O. Box 3792
Bartlesville, OK 74006

housewifeclass@gmail.com
www.housewifeclass.com
@housewifeclass

Ordering Information:

U.S. trade bookstores and wholesalers, please contact HWC Press. Special discounts are available on quantity purchase by corporations, association, educators, and others.

www.ingramcontent.com/pod-product-compliance
Lightning Source LLC
Chambersburg PA
CBHW060810270326
41928CB00002B/46